Gl

The 5 Ingredient — or less — KETOGENIC INSTANT Pot Cookbook

Get Lean & Healthy With Mouth-watering Breakfast, Lunch, Dinner, Soup & Dessert Recipes

Text Copyright © GEN GALE

All rights reserved. No part of this guide may be reproduced in any form without permission in writing from the publisher except in the case of brief quotations embodied in critical articles or reviews.

Legal & Disclaimer

The information contained in this book and its contents is not designed to replace or take the place of any form of medical or professional advice; and is not meant to replace the need for independent medical, financial, legal or other professional advice or services, as may be required. The content and information in this book has been provided for educational and entertainment purposes only.

The content and information contained in this book has been compiled from sources deemed reliable, and it is accurate to the best of the Author's knowledge, information and belief. However, the Author cannot guarantee its accuracy and validity and cannot be held liable for any errors and/or omissions. Further, changes are periodically made to this book as and when needed. Where appropriate and/or necessary, you must consult a professional (including but not limited to your doctor, attorney, financial advisor or such other professional advisor) before using any of the suggested remedies, techniques, or information in this book.

Upon using the contents and information contained in this book, you agree to hold harmless the Author from and against any damages, costs, and expenses, including any legal fees potentially resulting from the application of any of the information provided by this book. This disclaimer applies to any loss, damages or injury caused by the use and application, whether directly or indirectly, of any advice or information presented, whether for breach of contract, tort, negligence, personal injury, criminal intent, or under any other cause of action.

You agree to accept all risks of using the information presented inside this book.

You agree that by continuing to read this book, where appropriate and/or necessary, you shall consult a professional (including but not limited to your doctor, attorney, or financial advisor or such other advisor as needed) before using any of the suggested remedies, techniques, or information in this book.

Table of Contents

Introduction 7

Chapter 1: Relationship between Instant Pot and Keto Meals 9

Ketogenic Instant Pot - Breakfast 10

    Easy Keto Egg Frittata 11

    Easy Keto Egg Cups 13

    Korean Steamed Eggs 15

    Squash Spaghetti Noodles w/ Parmesan Cheese and Lemon Juice
.... 17

    Honey Glazed Ham and Cheese Sandwich 19

    Crust-less Meat Lovers Quiche 21

    Jalapeno Popper Omelet in a Jar 23

    Low-Carb Lasagna 25

Chapter 2: Meals-In-Five-Or-Less on a Keto Diet 27

Ketogenic Instant Pot – Lunch 29

    Jalapeno Popper Chicken Casserole 29

    Sausage and Kale 31

    Ketogenic Stroganoff 32

    Curried Chicken with Instant Lemon 33

    Whole Chicken 34

    Garlic Butter Chicken 35

    Shredded Chicken 36

    Beef Short Ribs 37

    Easy Hawaiian BBQ Meatballs 38

    Oxtail Recipe 39

    Lamb Stew 40

- Pot Luck Meatballs ... 41
  - Healthy Mississippi Pot Roast ... 42
- Ketogenic Instant Pot - Dinner ... 43
  - Homemade Pork Verde ... 44
  - Turnip Green ... 45
  - Turkey Breast ... 46
  - Low Carb Ground Beef Shawarma ... 48
  - Mama's Instant Pot Bean-less Chili Keto Beef ... 50
  - Mexican Chicken Pollo Con Salsa Rojo ... 52
  - Braised Beef Pot Roast ... 54
  - Easy Turkey Keto ... 56
  - Curry Beef Stew ... 57
  - Pork Chops ... 59
  - Easy Keto Beef Pot Roast ... 61
  - Cauliflower "Mac" and "Cheese" ... 63
- Healthy Instant Pot Soup ... 64
  - Low Carb Taco Soup ... 64
  - Low-Carb Cauliflower Soup ... 66
  - Low Carb Ham and Bean Soup ... 68
  - Chicken Mushroom Soup ... 70
  - Low Carb Keto Chicken Noodle Soup ... 72
  - Asparagus Soup ... 73
  - Chicken Soup ... 74
  - Quick Onion Soup ... 75
  - Broccoli Cheddar Soup ... 77
  - Bone Broth ... 78
- Instant Pot Dessert Recipes ... 79

Creme Brulee 79

Spiced Cider 81

Ricotta Lemon Cheesecake 82

Coconut Yogurt 84

Low Carb Peanut Butter Chocolate Cheesecake 86

Baked Apples 87

BONUS: 5 Day Ultimate Ketogenic Meal Plan for Rapid Fat Loss 88

Breakfast Recipes 89

Cheesy Jalapeno Egg Muffins 89

Coconut Flour Waffles 91

Low-Carb Breakfast Patties 92

Cheesy Spinach and Mushroom Quiche 94

Sausage and Spinach Mini Cups 96

Lunch Recipes 98

Stir-Fried Shrimps with Asparagus and Snap Pea 98

Honey-Soy Sesame Chicken 100

Mongolian Beef 101

Chicken and Broccoli Stir-Fry 103

Salmon Fillets with Curry Sauce and Cucumbers 105

Dinner Recipes 107

Chicken Gumbo 107

Oven-Baked Spinach and Quinoa 109

Tomato-Mushroom Chicken Casserole 111

Black Bean and Chickpea Soup with Chorizo 113

Lemon-Peppered Prawns 115

Conclusion 116

Check out Other Best Selling eBooks 117

Introduction

Trying out a new diet can be exciting but at the same time stressing. There are all these things you will need to avoid, eat more or simply add to your existing meals. Sometimes changing to a new diet can be as dramatic as requiring you to clean out your entire kitchen cabinet and buy new ingredients or as flawless as just buying one or two new ingredients.

The Ketogenic or "Keto" diet as it's popularly known is a diet that has been slowly gaining momentum. It is a high-fat diet that is low in carbohydrates and moderate in protein. It provides an almost perfect macro-nutrient ratio which makes it easy for the body to switch effortlessly from using fat to using carbohydrates.

The human body is highly dependent on both fat and carbohydrates for energy (fuel). The thing that's fascinating about the Keto diet is that it can encourage the body to burn fat rapidly. Scientists have for many years proven that fat is solely responsible for weight gain. And weight gain is associated to multiple illnesses including obesity and epilepsy in children and type 2 diabetes amongst others.

There are lots of benefits of a Ketogenic diet, the most prominent being it's fat-building properties. A consistent diet of foods with protein and high fat means that your body will start burning fat as opposed to burning proteins. Consequently, fat starts being converted to ketone bodies and fatty acids by the liver. The source of energy for your body becomes ketone body which is different from the use of glucose from carbohydrates in the traditional diet.

A lot of people think that the Keto diet is simple for people who are interested in losing weight. On the contrary, this type of diet that includes heart-healthy fats like fish, olive oil and nuts, and that limits sugars and processed grains can reduce or eliminate your risk of heart diseases. There are intense keto diets where only 5 percent of the diet comes from carbs, 20 percent is from protein and 75 percent is from fat. But even a modified version of this which involves consciously choosing foods low in carbohydrate and high in healthy fats is good enough.

Chapter 1: Relationship between Instant Pot and Keto Meals

While cooking keto is exciting, sometimes you lack the energy to make a complicated meal. An instant pot can, therefore, be your best friend in your keto kitchen. This is because it will reduce your cooking time to under an hour in most cases while at the same time demand very little effort from you. And you'll have less to clean up since there is only one pot being used in most cases.

A lot of people are concerned about cooking in a pressure cooker. People ask, is it safe? Is it healthy? How easy is it? Using an instant pot can actually make your foods healthier. One study that was done using broccoli discovered that 90% of vitamin C was retained on the broccoli when cooked on an instant pot while boiling reduced the amount to 66% and steaming reduced to 78%.

These findings are no surprise because when you cook using an instant pot you will use far less water compared to other methods, and a lot of water is what is credited for loss of minerals (water soluble).

Cooking with a pressure cooker is fun and safe. You will find tips on choosing the best pressure cooker and why the instant pot is the best at the end of the book on how to use your instant pot for the best results.

Ketogenic Instant Pot - Breakfast

The truth of the matter is that there is very little to work with for breakfast on keto. And because a lot of people feel satiated on a low-carb diet, they lose the appetite for morning meals. If you're amongst the group of people who don't feel hungry at the beginning of the day, you can skip breakfast and wait for the next meal.

For people who need a good breakfast to perform better during the day, taking a cereal like a majority of people is not a good idea. The reason a lot of people resort to cereal is that they are in a hurry and this is the easiest food to make. But with the following healthy keto recipes that can be made using an instant pot, you no longer have an excuse for a boring breakfast.

Easy Keto Egg Frittata

TOTAL TIME: 1 HR 40 MINUTES

SERVINGS: 4

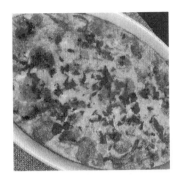

4 eggs

1 cup half and half

10 ounce canned green chilies

1 cup shredded cheese of any type

¼ chopped cilantro

1. Cut the canned chilies into small pieces
2. Beat eggs in a bowl and add half a cup of the shredded cheese, 1 cup half and half and green chilies. You can also add ¼ to ½ tsp. salt to taste if desired.
3. Pour the mixture into the generously greased pan and cover it with a foil.
4. In your instant pot, add two cups of water and place a trivet. Place the covered pot on top of the trivet.
5. Cook at high pressure for 20 minutes then for the next 10 minutes allow for natural release before you manually release the remaining pressure.
6. Evenly distribute the remaining half cup of shredded cheese on top of the tart and put it under a hot broiler. Leave it for five minutes or until you see the cheese bubbling and brown.

7. Remove and serve when hot. Serve with a salad on the side.

This recipe is for 4, so if you are making this for more people or for people with larger appetites, you can add more eggs and other ingredients. **Also, you can add other spices like 1 tsp. smoked paprika, hot paprika or oregano** *and add it to the grated cheese instead of the chilies. If you don't have half and half you can substitute it with crème Fraiche.*

Per Serving:

Calories: 110 kcal | **Fat:** 6g | **Carbs:** 1g | **Protein:** 7g

Easy Keto Egg Cups

It is a portable breakfast, which means that if you don't like eating early in the morning you can carry them to the office and warm in a microwave and you have your instant breakfast right away!

TOTAL TIME: 1 HR 10 MINUTES

SERVINGS: 4

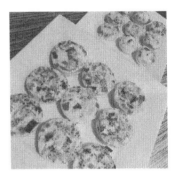

2 eggs

1 cup of cheese

¼ cup half and half

1 cup diced vegetables (mushrooms, onions, tomatoes, bell peppers etc.)

2 Tsps. chopped cilantro (or other herbs)

1. Beat the two eggs in a bowl.
2. Chop vegetables and add them to the eggs.
3. Add the half and half, cup of cheese, cilantro (or other herbs), salt, and pepper.
4. Divide the mixture into four parts in ½ pint wide mouth jars or any other suitable container.
5. Cover the containers so that water would not get into the eggs.
6. Pour two cups of water in your instant pot and place a trivet inside.

7. Place the jars on top of the trivet and cover the instant pot. Cook for five minutes at high pressure and then release the pressure manually.

8. Serve, or bring it out as a portable breakfast!

PER SERVING:

Calories: 90 kcal | **Fat:** 4g | **Carbs:** 3g | **Protein:** 7g

Korean Steamed Eggs

TOTAL TIME: 5 MINUTES

SERVINGS: 1

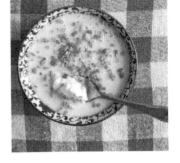

1 large egg

1/3 cup cold water

1 tsp. Chopped scallions

Pinch of garlic powder, pepper, and salt

Pinch of sesame seeds

1. Beat eggs in a small bowl and mix with water
2. Use a fine mesh strainer to strain the egg mixture into a heatproof bowl.
3. Ad all the other ingredients in the egg mixture and put aside.
4. Add one cup of water to the instant pot's inner pot.
5. Place the steamer basket or trivet inside the pot.
6. Place the bowl with the egg mixture on the steamer basket or trivet.
7. Close the instant pot tightly with the lid and close the vent valve
8. Use manual setting on "high" and cook for 5 minutes.
9. Quick release the pressure when the timer goes off.
10. Serve immediately with bread.

Recipe Note: *Although this recipe is designed for only one person, you can add eggs and other* **ingredients** *according to the number of people you're serving.*

PER SERVING:

Calories: 92 kcal | **Fat:** 5g | **Carbs:** 1.5g | **Protein:** 7g

Squash Spaghetti Noodles w/ Parmesan Cheese and Lemon Juice

TOTAL TIME: 10 MINUTES

SERVINGS: 6

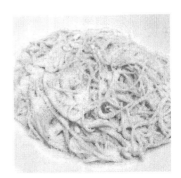

1 Pack of 2lb medium spaghetti squash

1 cup water

2 cloves Garlic

4 tbsp. Grated Parmesan cheese

Juice of 1/2 lemon

1. Cut spaghetti squash crosswise in half.
2. Core the squash to remove the seeds.
3. Place the trivet inside the instant pot and add one cup of water.
4. Arrange the squash halves on the steamer insert with the cut-side up. Cover the pot with the lid cover. Cook for about 7 minutes in high pressure. Press the manual button or pressure cook of the instant pot and hold the plus (+) or minus (-) sign button until you hit '7' on the display button.
5. Remove the lid cover and tip over the content to drain the liquid. Check by poking the squash using a fork. See to it that the squash is tender and temptingly delicious.
6. Take your squash halves out of the pot and shred using a fork. You now have your instant squash spaghetti noodles.

7. Ready your spaghetti noodles and the rest of the ingredients. Press SAUTE function button and let the pot heat up for 1-2 minutes, then add the olive oil and garlic, and stir for 30 seconds until it turns golden brown and smells good.

8. Add the noodles and drizzle with lemon juice. Mix gently with the flavored oil and garlic for 20-30 seconds. This is to coat the noodles with the flavored oil and to heat them up slightly but not overcook them. Season with salt and serve.

PER SERVING:

Calories: 230 kcal | **Fat:** 3g | **Carbs:** 40g | **Protein:** 10g

Honey Glazed Ham and Cheese Sandwich

The debate over cheese on a keto diet is one that doesn't seem to have a conclusion. If you're not comfortable eating cheese while on keto then you can substitute it with eggs for this easy instant pot honey glazed ham sandwich breakfast.

TOTAL TIME: 15 MINUTES

SERVINGS: 4

1 Boneless Quarter of ham (6-7 lbs. fully cooked)

1 cup brown sugar

½ cup honey

1 Tsp. Ground Cloves

4 Tbsp. natural pineapple Juice with titbits

1. Pour 1 cup of water in the instant pot in preparation for the ham.
2. Place the trivet or wire rack on top of the water.
3. Slice the ham evenly on a cutting board.
4. Construct a foil package and place the ham slices inside it.
5. Place the brown sugar across the top of the ham in an even distribution and dazzle the honey across the brown sugar.
6. Sprinkle with clove and add the pineapple juice and titbits.

7. Close the foil package and cover the instant pot with its lid.

8. Cook on manual for 10 minutes and then quickly release the steam.

9. Split low-carb buns, warm biscuit or low-carb bread and top each half bottom with a slice of ham and a slice of cheese or egg slices cover with the top half of the bread, biscuit or bun.

10. Serve with tea or place the sandwich on a foil-lined cookie sheet and carry to work.

Recipe Note: *To customize the recipe you can decrease or increase the sugar and honey. Be careful when opening the foil from the instant pot as it can easily burn you. Bread is not a keto-friendly food, you can, however, use low carb bread or buns like cloud bread.*

PER SERVING:

Calories: 350 kcal | **Fat:** 15g | **Carbs:** 30g | **Protein:** 20g

Crust-less Meat Lovers Quiche

Easy to cook and filling breakfast to start off meat lovers' on a good note.

TOTAL TIME: 30 MINUTES

SERVINGS: 6

6 eggs

4 slices bacon cooked & crumbled

1 cup of sausage or ½ cup ham

2 large green onions, chopped

1 cup of cheese

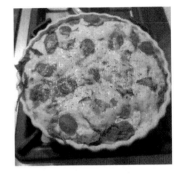

1. Place a metal trivet on your instant pot and add 1 cup of water
2. Whisk the eggs together in a large bowl and add half cup of milk, (or water) pepper, salt, and any other spice.
3. In a 1-quart well-greased soufflé dish, add the bacon, sausage (or/and ham), the two green onions and the cheese. Alternatively, you can place a foil sling on the dish before adding the meats.
4. Pour the egg mixture on top of the meat and stir.
5. Cover the soufflé dish loosely with an aluminium foil and place it inside your instant pot on top of the trivet.
6. Secure the lid and cook for 30 minutes in "High Pressure" setting. Wait for 10 minutes after the timer beeps and then quick release the pressure.

7. Open the lid carefully and remove the foil. You can then sprinkle your quiche with extra broil and cheese until it is slightly brown and then serve when hot.

Recipe Note: *This meal can serve 6, but you can modify it accordingly to fit the number of people you want to serve.*

PER SERVING:

Calories: 103 kcal | **Fat:** 6g | **Carbs:** 6g | **Protein:** 7g

Jalapeno Popper Omelet in a Jar

If you are too busy to devote a lot of time towards a healthy breakfast, this low-carb keto can be whipped up in less than 10 minutes.

TOTAL TIME: 10 MINUTES

SERVINGS: 4

12 large eggs beaten (pasture raised, organic)

1 cup of shredded cheddar cheese

8 slices of bacon chopped

4 medium-sized jalapeno peppers chopped and seeded

¼ cup of heavy cream

1. Prepare the jars by spraying them with avocado oil spray.
2. Cooked chopped bacon over medium heat in a skillet until crispy and then remove the bacon from fat and set it aside.
3. Cook the chopped jalapeños in the bacon until soft (1-2 mins) and then remove and set aside.
4. Beat the eggs in a bowl and add the heavy cream until properly mixed. Fold in the shredded cheddar cheese and the bacon and add extra pepper and salt to your taste.
5. Divide the mixture into four jars.
6. Place the trivet inside your pressure cooker and add 2 cups of water. Place the jars on a rack and cover with the

7. Cook on "high pressure" setting for 7 minutes and then allow the pressure to release naturally.

8. Serve immediately when hot or keep in the refrigerator and reheat when desired. It can only last for 1 week inside the fridge.

Recipe Notes: *You can cook this for 5 minutes for a softer egg or for immediate consumption. After it has naturally depressurized, you can stir to prevent the hot cooked egg from solidifying. The number of jalapeños and other spices you add will depend on how spicy you want your omelettes to be.*

PER SERVING:

Calories: 120 kcal | **Fat:** 7g | **Carbs:** 6g | **Protein:** 15g

Low-Carb Lasagna

TOTAL TIME: 25 MINUTES

SERVINGS: 8

1 lb. ground beef

8 ounces sliced mozzarella

1 ½ cup ricotta cheese

I large egg

1 small onion

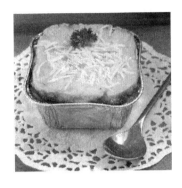

1. Brown the ground beef on sauté setting. Add onions, or you can choose to add 2 cloves of minced garlic.

2. When the meat is still brown, combine the eggs and 1 cup of ricotta cheese in a small bowl, you can also add other types of cheese like parmesan cheese.

3. You can then remove half of the meat sauce and replace it with marinara sauce.

4. Sprinkle a layer of mozzarella cheese but reserve some for the final layer.

5. Spread the remaining ricotta cheese on top of the mozzarella.

6. Loosely cover the lasagna bowl with a loose aluminium foil to prevent water that will result from condensation from dripping onto the cheese.

7. On your instant pot, place the trivet and add a cup of water. Place the lasagna on top of the trivet and cover the pot.

8. Cook for 8-10 minutes at "high pressure" setting.

9. Quick release the steam removes the bowl of lasagna and add any extra cheese on top cover and let it sit for the cheese to melt.

10. Spoon the lasagna into table bowls and serve.

PER SERVING:

Calories: 339 kcal | **Fat:** 28g | **Carbs:** 9g | **Protein:** 38g

Chapter 2: Meals-In-Five-Or-Less on a Keto Diet

A lot of people choose to eat in a 6 or 8-hour time lapse. This usually means skipping breakfast so that they only have lunch and dinner. A secret for getting into ketosis faster is to burn off stored glycogen through fasting. Although the ketogenic diet or keto meal plans don't necessarily encourage this, skipping lunch or one of the other meals while on the keto diet could actually be extremely helpful.

There are however people who feel great on breakfast and lunch and are usually too tired in the night to make dinner. If this is the case for you then you will benefit from these easy keto meal recipes that only require you to have a maximum of five **ingredients**.

What makes switching to a keto diet easy is the fact that many foods recommended in this diet are foods that you're already enjoying. The only foods that you will be excluded are those high in fats including:

    i.   Pasta

    ii.   Bread

    iii. Noodles

    iv.   Rice

    v.   Pastries and Sweets

    vi.   Cereals

    vii. Juices and Sodas

    viii. Most fruits

So basically, anything made out of sugar or flour will have to find its way out of your kitchen. Thankfully in this 21st-century world, there is always an alternative and you can make a keto version of the high-carb dishes you were enjoying on a non-keto diet. You will simply need to substitute some of the **ingredients**, for instance, use almond or coconut flour in place of regular flour, and use sweetener like a stevia as a substitute for sugar.

The secret of a good lunch in a keto diet is to focus on all of the tasty and healthy food options you enjoy instead of focusing on all the foods you cannot have. Is it not great that the keto diet puts on the table all meats and you can prepare them in basically any type of way you like and using all types of seasoning? You can eat chicken, turkey, beef, pork, tuna, salmon, bison and even kangaroo or snake if you like.

Eggs are also a good option on this diet and there are endless ways of preparing this for any meal. There are also a good number of vegetables you cannot go wrong with on a keto diet, especially the ones that are grown above ground.

Without further ado, let's get started with the ketogenic instant pot meals that can be prepared with just 5 ingredients or less.

Ketogenic Instant Pot – Lunch
Jalapeno Popper Chicken Casserole

This instant pot Jalapeno Popper Chicken Casserole is really just the adult version of mac and cheese, or a spiced up classic chicken chilly.

TOTAL TIME: 15 MINUTES

SERVINGS: 4

3 and 1/3 cups Boneless cook and dice chicken breasts

2 cups chicken broth/stock

3 jalapenos, 2 diced and one sliced

6 ounces challenge cream cheese, softened and cut into 1 inch pieces

1 cup cook and diced bacon

Half diced onion, 3 tsp minced garlic, 1 tsp cumin, ¼ tsp black pepper
1/8 tsp salt & sugarless diced tomatoes (optional)

1. Combine chicken breast, jalapeno, half diced onion, 3 teaspoons minced garlic 1 teaspoon cumin, ¼ teaspoon black pepper, 1/8 tsp. salt, the chicken broth, and 10 ounces of sugarless diced tomatoes.

2. Lock the instant pot in place and seal the steam nozzle. Cook on "soup" setting for 10 minutes.

3. Stir in half of the bacon into the chicken in the instant pot and add the jalapeno and cream cheese.

4. Pour this into a greased casserole dish and cover with an aluminium foil.

5. Place the trivet inside the instant pot and add one cup of water.

6. Place the dish with casserole inside the pot and cook on warm for 3 minutes.

7. Remove the foil from the dish and sprinkle with some cheese, sliced jalapeno and bacon that was left.

Recipe Notes: *This recipe is simply a modified version of a backed chicken and bacon casserole. You can use either canned or fresh jalapeno. If you want to freeze this meal for serving later you should re-adjust the Instructions for its preparation.*

PER SERVING:

Calories: 130 kcal | **Fat:** 5g | **Carbs:** 16g | **Protein:** 10g

Sausage and Kale

This recipe, like most others in the instant pot keto recipes for lunch, can be made for either a quick lunch or dinner. The instant pot sausage and kale is in fact almost like a cheat recipe in the fact that it virtually needs no type of preparation and can be on the table in less than 10 minutes.

TOTAL TIME: 10 MINUTES

SERVINGS: 4

4 smoked sausages

5 and ½ cups chopped kale

¼ cup water

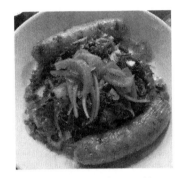

1. Pour all the **ingredients** into your instant pot's inner liner and cook on "high pressure" setting for 4 minutes.

2. All for natural pressure release for 5 minutes and then quick release the remaining pressure.

3. Serve when hot.

PER SERVING:

Calories: 223 kcal | **Fat:** 6g | **Carbs:** 3g | **Protein:** 12g

Ketogenic Stroganoff

TOTAL TIME: 30 MINUTES

SERVINGS: 4

Low carb noodles or Cauliflower Rice

1-lb pork strips or beef stew meat

1 and ½ cups chopped mushrooms

1/3 cup sour cream

1 Tsp. oil

Worcestershire Sauce & Salt (optional)

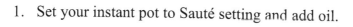

1. Set your instant pot to Sauté setting and add oil.
2. Add the pork strips or beef stew meat, the mushrooms, 1 tablespoon Worcestershire sauce and a teaspoon of salt. Top this up with ¾ cup of water.
3. Cook on "high pressure" setting for 20 minutes and then allow for natural pressure release for 10 minutes before you release the rest of the pressure.
4. Add 1/3 cup of sour cream.
5. Once you are satisfied with the thickness, serve with low carb noodles or cauliflower rice.

PER SERVING:

Calories: 321 kcal | **Fat:** 8g | **Carbs:** 8g | **Protein:** 17g

Curried Chicken with Instant Lemon

TOTAL TIME: 4 HR

SERVINGS: 6

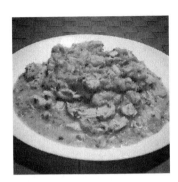

1 can Coconut Milk (full fat)

1/4 cup Lemon juice

1 tsp Turmeric

6 Pcs. Chicken breasts or thighs

1 tbsp. Curry Spice

1. Set your instant pot on high heat.
2. Add all ingredients and set on the manual setting.
3. Secure the vent sealing and cover. Set the timer for about 4 hours.
4. Serve hot!

PER SERVING:

Calories: 321 kcal | **Fat:** 15g | **Carbs:** 14g | **Protein:** 20g

Whole Chicken

TOTAL TIME: 50 MINUTES

SERVINGS: 6

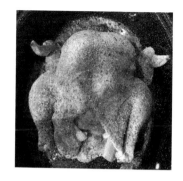

3lb whole Chicken

1 whole Yellow or Red Onion

1 tbsp. Coconut Oil

1 cup Water

1. Pour a cup of water in your instant pot and lay the steam rack inside it.
2. Heat coconut oil in a large skillet and add the chicken. Allow it to sear for about a minute on each side. Remove from heat.
3. Arrange the chicken on the top of the steam rack of the instant pot. Secure the lid and set it to Chicken (high pressure) before adjusting the time. Assign 6 minutes for every pound of chicken. Add 2 minutes to the total cooking time.
4. Allow steam to release for about 20 minutes. Serve while hot.

Recipe Notes: This is a simple chicken recipe that you can customize however you like and serve with your favorite vegetables. You can season the chicken by placing a whole lemon inside it for a tangy citrus flavor, season with crushed peppercorns, or with dried or fresh herbs.

PER SERVING:

Calories: 236 kcal | **Fat:** 10g | **Carbs:** 0g | **Protein:** 20g

Garlic Butter Chicken

TOTAL TIME: 40 MINUTES

SERVING: 4

4 Pcs. Chicken breast, chopped or whole

10 cloves garlic, peeled and diced

1/4 cup turmeric ghee (or mix 1 tsp. turmeric with regular ghee)

Salt to taste

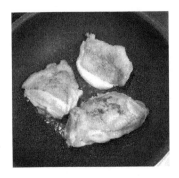

1. Place chicken breasts inside the instant pot.
2. Add the turmeric ghee, garlic and salt.
3. Set the instant pot on high pressure for about 35 minutes, following the instruction specifically on securing the valve and lid cover and in releasing pressure when cooking time is over.
4. Shred chicken breasts while still in the pot and serve with additional ghee when needed.

PER SERVING:

Calories: 301 kcal | **Fat:** 14g | **Carbs:** 1g | **Protein:** 28g

Shredded Chicken

Shredded chicken has versatile uses for making tacos, salads to last-minute stir-fry. You can even carry this to work for lunch by making a chicken salad sandwich using chipotle mayo.

TOTAL TIME: 30 MINUTES
SERVINGS: 8

4 lbs. Chicken breasts
1/2 tsp. Black pepper
1/2 cup chicken broth or water
1 tsp. Salt

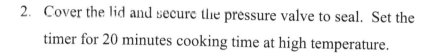

1. Place ingredients in the instant pot.
2. Cover the lid and secure the pressure valve to seal. Set the timer for 20 minutes cooking time at high temperature.
3. Once the cooking time is complete, turn the valve venting to release pressure. When all pressure managed to escape, you can then open the lid.
4. Place chicken on a platter or cutting board and shred to pieces using forks.
5. Store chicken in an airtight container along with the liquid. This will keep the chicken constantly moist.

PER SERVING:

Calories: 252 kcal | **Fat:** 8g | **Carbs:** 5g | **Protein:** 38g

Beef Short Ribs

TOTAL TIME: 55 HR

SERVINGS: 8

2 lbs. Beef short ribs, boneless

1 pc. Onion, diced

3 tbsps. Tamari sauce

2 tbsps. White wine or vodka

Salt to taste

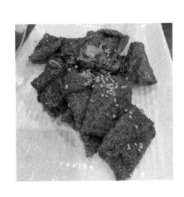

1. Place all ingredients in the instant pot.
2. Press the button indicating Meat/Stew and set the timer for 45 minutes.
3. Wait until the cooking time is over and allow it to vent until pressure is totally released'.
4. Serve.

PER SERVING:

Calories: 164 kcal | **Fat:** 6g | **Carbs:** 0g | **Protein:** 25g

Easy Hawaiian BBQ Meatballs

TOTAL TIME: 20 MINUTES

SERVINGS: 4

8-Oz of crushed pineapple

12 Oz of BBQ sauce

1 bag of frozen meatballs

1. Place meatballs into the instant pot and cover meatballs with BBQ sauce.
2. Add crushed pineapples and stir gently. Secure the vent to seal and close the lid cover of the instant pot. Put to manual setting and set the timer for 6 minutes cooking. Once the time is over, release the pressure quickly. Wait until all the pressure are released before trying to open the cover of the instant pot.
3. Serve and enjoy!

PER SERVING:

Calories: 155 kcal | **Fat:** 8g | **Carbs:** 5g | **Protein:** 15g

Oxtail Recipe

TOTAL TIME: 7 HR

SERVINGS: 6

3.5 lbs. Of Oxtail

1-2 sprigs each of rosemary and thyme

2 tbsp. lemon juice

2 1/2 L. of water or bone broth

Salt and pepper to taste

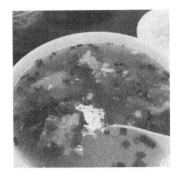

1. Preheat a greased Dutch oven over medium-high heat. Pat dry using paper towels and then season with salt and pepper. Place oxtails in a large pot and cook for about 10 minutes to brown all sides. When meat turns brown, transfer to the instant pot and set it to slow cook for about 4 hours.
2. Add thyme and bay leaves secured in a cheesecloth for easy removal once cooked.
3. Add the water or broth with lemon juice and bring to boil. Reduce heat to low and cover with the lid. Leave it to simmer for 3 hours or until the meat becomes tender and falls off the bones. Vent to reduce pressure before opening.
4. Discard the cloth and serve the dish in a bowl.

PER SERVING:

Calories: 148 kcal | **Fat:** 7g | **Carbs:** 0g | **Protein:** 17.5g

Lamb Stew

TOTAL TIME: 40 MINUTES

SERVINGS: 5

2 lbs. Lamb stew meat

6 cloves Garlic

1 large Yellow onion

1 pc. Acorn squash

3 pcs. Large Carrots

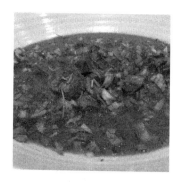

1. Start by peeling the acorn squash, core, and cut into cubes. Also, peel carrots and cut into thick rounds. Likewise, peel the onions and cut in half then cut crosswise to form half-moons. If you want your veggies to be firmer, cut them bigger.

2. Place ingredients in the instant pot and set to soup/stew setting. Cook for 35 minutes.

3. When done, carefully release the pressure before unlocking the lid.

4. Serve and enjoy!

PER SERVING:

Calories: 150 kcal | **Fat:** 6g | **Carbs:** 0g | **Protein:** 23g

Pot Luck Meatballs

TOTAL TIME: 15 MINUTES

SERVINGS: 6

1 jar of Grape Jelly

1 Bottle of BBQ Sauce (12-14 oz.)

2 bags of 20-Oz. Meatballs

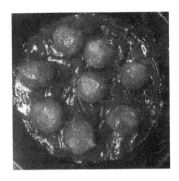

1. Throw in all ingredients inside your instant pot. Mix well and secure the lid.
2. Set to manual mode for 9 minutes and when the timer stops, simply open the vent valve to release the pressure.
3. When the pin goes down, you can now open the lid cover and your meatballs are ready to serve.

PER SERVING:

Calories: 155 kcal | **Fat:** 8g | **Carbs:** 0g | **Protein:** 15g

Healthy Mississippi Pot Roast

TOTAL TIME: 1 HR 10 MINUTES

SERVINGS: 8

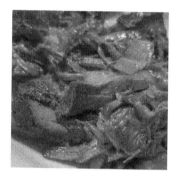

3-4 lbs. of chuck roast

1/2 stick of butter

1 packet of ranch seasoning mix

1/2 jar Pepperoncini including the juice

1 cup of beef broth

1. Start by seasoning your meat with half of the ranch seasoning mix package content. Allow it to sit for 20 minutes
2. Place beef broth in the instant pot followed by chuck roast. Then add the rest of the ranch package content. Top it with butter.
3. Secure the lid and set the pot in manual mode for 22 minutes for every pound of roast you work with.
4. When cooking time is over as the timer goes off, release the pressure naturally for 10-15 minutes. When it's over, open the valve and allow the remaining pressure to come out.
5. Lastly, open the lid and the tender roast is now ready for serving.

PER SERVING:

Calories: 300 kcal | **Fat:** 17g | **Carbs:** 3g | **Protein:** 32g

Ketogenic Instant Pot - Dinner

Plenty of people who are on a diet or are trying to lose weight usually thinks that breakfast and lunch are the most important meals of the day and that it's okay to skip dinner. Meal patterns that don't stress the importance of dinner are restricting because let's face it; most of us are extremely busy building our career. This meaning we would get caught up with work and therefore have insufficient time in the morning for a proper breakfast, having been able to only grab a bagel or sandwich.

So, if there is a good moment to enjoy a good meal, it's dinner time. Besides, dinner is also the only time you can get to spend with your family and enjoy each other's company. The following recipes with less than five **ingredients** are so simple that you won't have to stress over making dinner after a hectic day at work.

Homemade Pork Verde

TOTAL TIME: 50 MINUTES

SERVINGS: 10

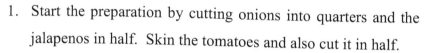

3 lbs. of Tomatillos

1 pc. Garlic, minced

2 lbs. of Pork Chops, diced

1 large onion, sliced

1 large jalapeno

1. Start the preparation by cutting onions into quarters and the jalapenos in half. Skin the tomatoes and also cut it in half.
2. Roast the tomatoes in the oven. To roast your veggies, set your oven on broil and place the tomatoes in the oven until their tops turned semi-black. Once done, take it out of the oven and blend using a blender till it turns into a sauce-like mixture.
3. Place the sauce and diced pork into the instant pot and set to manual cooking for 6 minutes. When the pressure cooker beeps, naturally release the pressure for about 10 minutes. Open the valve and release the remaining steam.
4. Serve with a bowl and enjoy!

Recipe Notes: *I prefer buying pork stew meat that is pre-cut into cubes. You could choose to cut a pork shoulder into cubes or cook it in large chunks instead but it will take longer to cook!*

PER SERVING:

Calories: 192 kcal | **Fat:** 8g | **Carbs:** 6g | **Protein:** 24g

Turnip Green

TOTAL TIME: 22 MINUTES

SERVINGS: 4

16 oz. Turnip Greens

Bacon bits or ham pieces

Salt pepper to taste

2 cups of water or chicken broth

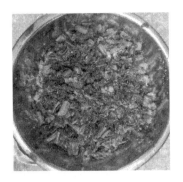

1. Wash and drain your veggies well. Place them inside the instant pot and add your chicken broth or water.
2. Top it with ham or bacon and season with salt and pepper to taste.
3. Secure the lid cover of the instant pot and set the timer for 12 minutes. When the timer is up, let it release pressure naturally for 10 minutes. Open the valve and allow the remaining pressure to get fully released.

PER SERVING:

Calories: 50 kcal | **Fat:** 3g | **Carbs:** 4g | **Protein:** 3g

Turkey Breast

TOTAL TIME: 1 HR

SERVINGS: 1

1 Turkey Breast

3 tsp. corn starch

3 tsp. of poultry seasoning

1 can of 16-Oz. Chicken broth

3 tsp. of garlic

Salt and pepper to taste (optional)

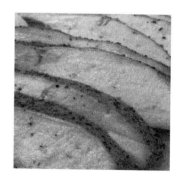

1. Season the turkey with garlic, poultry seasoning, salt, and pepper. Prepare your instant pot by placing the trivet inside the pot and add the chicken broth
2. Place the turkey with the big side up inside the cooker. Secure by sewing the vent and lid and set to pressure cook for 30 minutes. When the time is over, turn off the pressure cooker and allow the pressure to be naturally released.
3. While releasing the pressure, turn the oven to 450 degrees Fahrenheit to make sure that the skin will be crispy.
4. After 10-15 minutes, simply let out the remaining pressure. Once the pressure is totally released, carefully transfer the turkey to a baking sheet and cook for another 10 minutes but make sure to watch that the skin of the turkey doesn't get burned. While the turkey is getting crispy, add corn starch to a cup of water and mix. Once it's well blended and becomes

milky in consistency, place it bac
However, remove the trivet from th

5. Mix it well to have a nice, delicious
6. When the turkey is done, take it ou
   out of the bone, slice, and place on
7. Serve and enjoy!

PER SERVING:

Calories: 118 kcal | **Fat:** 1.9g | **Carbs:** 4g

Low Carb Ground Beef Shawarma

This instant pot low carb ground beef Shawarma with vegetables is a flavor-filled, family friendly instant pot meal for a fast dinner for your family.

TOTAL TIME: 7 MINUTES

SERVINGS: 4

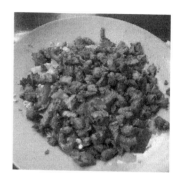

1-lb lean ground beef

2 tablespoons Shawarma mix

1 cup sliced onion

2 cups cubed cabbage

1 cup red peppers thickly sliced

Salt or pepper (optional)

1. Set your instant pot on "sauté". When it's hot, add ground beef and stir till it breaks into manageable chunks. You don't have to wait for it to fully brown before continuing with the recipe if the chunks have been broken.

2. Add all the **ingredients** and a teaspoon of salt or pepper to taste. Don't add any water since enough water will be released by the vegetables and meat.

3. Cook in an instant pot for 2 minutes. Allow for natural pressure release for 5 minutes and the quick release the remaining pressure.

4. Serve when hot.

Recipe Notes: *You can substitute the lean ground beef with any meat of your choice. Freezing is not recommended as the vegetables may get mushy when you reheat.*

PER SERVING:

Calories: 200 kcal | **Fat:** 15g | **Carbs:** 3g | **Protein:** 34g

Mama's Instant Pot Bean-less Chili Keto Beef

TOTAL TIME: 15 MINUTES

SERVINGS: 8

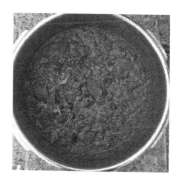

2 lbs. ground beef grass-fed or pork

1 cup chicken or beef broth for thinning

1 medium onion chopped (or ¼ cup onion flakes dried)

2 cloves minced garlic (or garlic powder 1 teaspoon)

5 Tsps. chili powder

1. Brown the ground beef on "sauté" setting on instant pot. Add chopped onion into the beef until brown.

2. When the beef is almost ready, add garlic & chili powder. Do not drain the fat from the ground beef.

3. Pour in one cup of chicken or beef broth and sugarless tomato sauce and paste if available without any stirring. This will ensure that the chilly does not burn when you start to pressure cook.

4. Cook on "high pressure" setting for 10 minutes. Leave it to release pressure naturally for 10 minutes and then quick release the pressure.

5. Check to see if the thickness is good for you. If you find it too watery after stirring put it back on the instant pot under sauté mode or an extra 5-10 minutes. Serve when hot.

6. Serve when hot.

Recipe Notes: *This recipe is best to eat on a day that you won't have any other meals or snacks all through, since its very filling. It can be served with sour cream, raw onion, cheese and some low carb "corn" bread. As for the added Mexican oregano in the instructions, I noticed that it makes so much difference in the flavor. You can customize this recipe any way you like as I do with most of my recipes. You could even try the recipe with "Carne picada" chopped beef and discover a whole new another flavor.*

PER SERVING:

Calories: 250 kcal | **Fat:** 17g | **Carbs:** 15g | **Protein:** 18g

Mexican Chicken Pollo Con Salsa Rojo

This fast, delicious instant pot chicken will change your view of cooking chicken meals for lunch. A lot of people only make chicken for dinner since they fear the amount of preparation that goes into making these meals. You can prepare this recipe within 10 minutes and in 25 minutes it will be ready for consumption.

TOTAL TIME: 25 MINUTES

SERVINGS: 3

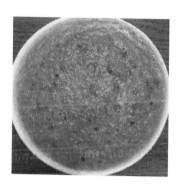

2 lbs. boneless, skinless chicken thighs cut into bite sizes

2 ounces pickled/ canned jalapenos

1 small onion, chopped

3 cloves ground garlic

1 and ½ Tsp. ground cumin

Chili Powder & Salt (optional)

1. Set the instant pot to "sauté" cooking mode.
2. As the instant pot is heating, coat the chicken thighs with cumin, 1 spoon chili powder and Tsp. of salt.
3. Pour 2 tsps. Of oil into the instant pot once it's hot and add the pieces of coated chicken and let it cook for 4-5 minutes. This will help the chicken bloom to their full flavor.

4. Add all the other ingredients to the chicken in the instant pot and cover.

5. Cook at "high pressure" setting and allow it to cook for 15 minutes then allow for natural pressure release for 10 minutes. Release the remaining pressure.

6. Serve as tacos by shredding the chicken pieces a bit more using a fork.

Recipe Notes: *You can replace the chicken in this recipe with pork. But that wouldn't be chicken pollo now, would it?*

PER SERVING:

Calories: 250 kcal | **Fat:** 5g | **Carbs:** 7g | **Protein:** 15g

Braised Beef Pot Roast

Pot roast is an excellent meal for dinner and has been popular with many families for generations. Yet many people shy away from this meal because they find it to be time-consuming. Here is a time-saving recipe that your whole family will love.

TOTAL TIME: 1 HR 30 MINUTES

SERVINGS: 12

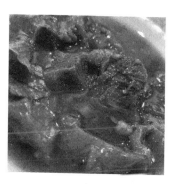

4-5-lb beef roast

2 tsp. garlic powder

2 Tsp. ghee or your favorite cooking fat like avocado oil

2tsp fine sea salt

Cracked black pepper (adds more flavor)

1. Press the sauté button on your Instant Pot and allow it some time to heat up; 2-3 minutes.

2. While the pot is heating up to the required temperature, season one side of the pot with half of the sea salt, garlic powder, and black pepper.

3. Add the ghee or avocado oil to the pot and place the roasted side of the beef roast into the bottom of the pot. Try to make sure that the maximum of the roast touches the bottom of the pot. Allow the roast to sear on one side, use the timer to ensure it boils for ten minutes.

4. Use the rest of the sea salt garlic powder and pepper to season the upward facing side. Flip the roast over after exactly ten minutes.

5. Press the "keep warm/cancel" button and cover the instant pot with the pressure release knob set to "sealing".

6. Set the timer to cook for 85 minutes

7. Let the Instant Pot release the steam without manually moving the pressure release knob. This should take 30 minutes to 1 hour. The lid will easily unlock once all the pressure is released.

8. You are now good to go! Scoop the roast out of the pot ensuring that you are leaving its liquid behind. Transfer the roast to your prepared serving pot. Enjoy the meal!

Recipe Notes: *Try serving this pot roast with your favorite roasted vegetables. You will lie to tell a story!*

PER SERVING:

Calories: 230 kcal | **Fat:** 6g | **Carbs:** 4g | **Protein:** 26g

Easy Turkey Keto

TOTAL TIME: 48 MINUTES

SERVINGS: 2

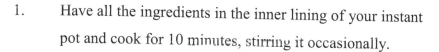

1.25 lbs. ground turkey or beef

One cup of sugar-free salsa Verde

1 tsp. salt and pepper to add taste

1tsp ground coriander

Red onion, cilantro, sour cream, avocado,

1 tsp. chopped scotch bonnet (optional)

Cheddar cheese, chopped chilly & habaneros (optional)

1. Have all the ingredients in the inner lining of your instant pot and cook for 10 minutes, stirring it occasionally.
2. Add the meat to the salsa; this will make it absorb the flavor while cooking. Do not brown the meat.
3. Garnish with any or all of the following; red onion, avocado, fried plantains, cilantro, fresh pineapple (finely chopped) and chopped habaneros.
4. Serve appropriate size which is 1 cup of average size. Enjoy the meal!

PER SERVING:

Calories: 275 kcal | **Fat:** 11g | **Carbs:** 13g | **Protein:** 32g

Curry Beef Stew

TOTAL TIME: 50 MINUTES

SERVINGS: 4

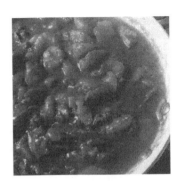

2.5 lbs. beef stew chunks (or a roasted beef chop into small cubes)

½ cup of chicken broth

14-ounce coconut milk

3 zucchinis, chopped

1-lb broccoli florets

2 tsp curry powder, 1 tsp garlic powder, Salt (optional)

1. All the ingredients except coconut milk in your instant pot. Add also 2 tablespoons of curry powder, 1 tablespoon of garlic powder and salt to taste.

2. Mix everything together. The goal here should be to keep the vegetables at the top and the beef at the bottom of the pot so that nothing is overcooked.

3. Cook on "high pressure" setting on your instant pot for 45 minutes. Quick release the pressure when the timer goes off.

4. After the stew is well cooked, add the coconut milk and stir. Taste and add extra salt if needed.

5. Serve in bowls when hot.

Recipe Notes: *No easier recipe for a tender and delicious beef stew. The zucchini and broccoli are only for keeping the carb count low, but you can add other vegetables if you wish.*

PER SERVING:

Calories: 490 kcal | **Fat:** 30g | **Carbs:** 8g | **Protein:** 40g

Pork Chops

TOTAL TIME: 30 MINUTES

SERVINGS: 4

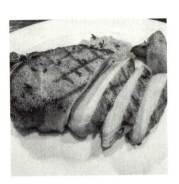

4 pork chops with bones or boneless

1 cup chicken broth

8 ounces mushrooms, chopped

2 tsp. coconut oil, divided

2 tsp. ghee or butter

Salt and pepper (optional)

1. Set your instant pot to warm.
2. Season the pork chops with salt and pepper (optional) on both sides.
3. Once the pot is hot, add 1 teaspoon of coconut oil.
4. Add in the pork chops ensuring that they're nicely seared. You can do it in two batches if you have a small or medium-sized instant pot. Sear on each side for roughly 2 minutes and then set them apart.
5. Add 1 teaspoon of coconut milk that was remaining.
6. Add the mushrooms and sauté for 2 more minutes before pouring in the chicken broth. If there are any brown bits sticking to the bottom of the instant pot scrap them.
7. Add in the pork chops and cover your instant pot.

8. Cook on high pressure setting for 10 minutes and then use the pressure valve to quick release the pressure.

9. You can then steam for about 5 minutes if there is too much sauce. Lastly, add ghee or butter and remove it from the heat.

10. Serve this pork chops with mushroom sauce on top and bacon roasted Brussels sprouts.

PER SERVING:

Calories: 241 kcal | **Fat:** 8g | **Carbs:** 8g | **Protein:** 22g

Easy Keto Beef Pot Roast

TOTAL TIME: 45 MINUTES

SERVINGS: 4

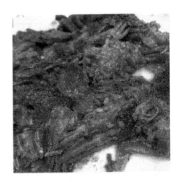

3 lbs. boneless beef roast

¼ cup balsamic vinegar

½ cup onion, chopped

1 tsp. ground pepper

¼ xanthan gum

Garlic powder, salt & pepper (optional)

1. Cut your chunk of roast into two pieces. Season with garlic powder, pepper, and salt on both sides.
2. Set your instant pot to sauté and let the roast brown on both sides.
3. Add ½ cup onion, ¼ cup balsamic vinegar and 1 cup water to the roast. Don't add the water directly onto the meat but rather to the sides so that it doesn't "wash" the flavor.
4. Cover the instant pot and cook on high pressure for 35 minutes.
5. Use a fork and a knife to cut the chunk of beef into manageable pieces. Remove any large pieces of fat and other unwanted parts.
6. Simmer the mixture for 10 minutes on sauté setting.

7. Add the Xanthium gum onto the meat in small bits as you observe the thickness.

8. Remove from the heat and serve hot in bowls.

Recipe Notes: You can serve this balsamic beef pot roast over cauliflower puree. You can garnish with freshly chopped parsley.

Cauliflower "Mac" and "Cheese"

TOTAL TIME: 30 MINUTES

SERVINGS: 4

2 cups cauliflower, riced

½ cup shredded sharp cheddar cheese

½ cup half and half

2 tablespoon cream cheese

Salt and pepper to taste

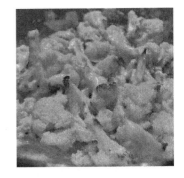

1. Mix all the ingredients together in a heatproof bowl
2. Cover the bowl with an aluminium foil
3. Pour 1 and ½ cups of water inside your instant pot and put the trivet inside. Place the covered pot on the trivet.
4. Set your instant pot on high pressure and allow for natural pressure release for 10 minutes.
5. Heat the oven broiler and broil the cauliflower until the cheese is bubbling and brown. Serve immediately.

Recipe Notes: The instructions may seem like you're making a quiche but the final product has a mac and cheese texture as opposed to a quiche texture.

PER SERVING:

Calories: 180 kcal | **Fat:** 8g | **Carbs:** 25g | **Protein:** 17g

Healthy Instant Pot Soup
Low Carb Taco Soup

TOTAL TIME: 15 MINUTES

SERVINGS: 8

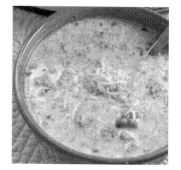

2-lb ground beef

32 ounces beef broth

8 ounces cream cheese

1 cup heavy cream

4 cloves garlic

Optional Toppings (optional)

Sliced black olives

Sour cream

Cheddar cheese

Sliced jalapeno peppers

1. Brown the ground beef with 4 cloves of garlic on a sauté setting. Drain the excess grease if there is any.
2. Stir in beef broth
3. Place the lid on the instant pot and cook on a "high pressure" setting for 5 minutes and then let it release pressure naturally for 10 minutes.
4. After all the pressure has been released, open the vent valve and add in cream cheese and heavy cheese.
5. Serve hot with the optional settings.

Recipe Note: *While toppings can make this recipe more versatile and add more flavor to the soup, be careful with these while on a strict keto diet. Also, avoid going overboard with tomatoes since they have natural sugars.*

PER SERVING:

Calories: 386 kcal | **Fat:** 30g | **Carbs:** 8g | **Protein:** 35g

Low-Carb Cauliflower Soup

TOTAL TIME: 5 MINUTES

SERVINGS: 4-6

3 cups chicken stock

1 small onion

4 ounces cream cheese cut into cubes

1 large head cauliflower

1 cup grated cheddar cheese

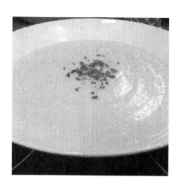

Optional Toppings

Sour cream

Extra grated sharp cheddar cheese

Thinly sliced green onions

8-10 strips bacon, cooked crisp and crumbled

1. Chop the small peeled onion into small pieces

2. Cut away the leaves of the cauliflower, and a part of the stem and chop the core into pieces after washing.

3. Under sauté, setting on your instant pot, melt butter and add onion. Let it cook for 2-3 minutes then add cauliflower, chicken stock, garlic powder, and salt. Replace the lid on the instant pot and cook under "high pressure" setting for 5 minutes. Quick release the pressure.

4. In a separate bowl add cream cheese cubes, half cup milk or half and half and grated sharp cheddar cheese. You can also add toppings like green onions, sour cream, and crumbled bacon.

5. Once it is safe to open the lid on your instant pot, confirm that the cauliflower is tender and then turn the setting to "keep warm" so that it simmers.

6. Puree the soup using a food processor or emersion blender. To make the soup thicker some more or add some more stock.

7. Add some cream cheese cubes, grated cheese and stir. And more half and half or milk and heat for 2 minutes. Add seasoning of salt and fresh ground black pepper to taste.

8. Serve hot with toppings that can be added to the table (green onion, crumbled bacon. Sour cream, grated cheese)

Recipe Note: *If this recipe ends up giving more soup than necessary, simply serve what is required and then freeze the rest.*

PER SERVING:

Calories: 131 kcal | **Fat:** 8g | **Carbs:** 9g | **Protein:** 5g

Low Carb Ham and Bean Soup

You probably know that ordinary beans are a no-no on a keto diet. But did you know that you can cheat this diet by having some great tasting low carb bean?

TOTAL TIME: 50 MINUTES

SERVINGS: 6

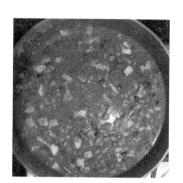

1 cup soaked dried black beans (will give 2 cups)

2 smoked ham hocks or 1 meaty ham bone

2 cups chopped ham

1 cup chopped onion

4 cloves minced garlic

1. Put all the ingredients in your instant pot. You can add a teaspoon of dried oregano, a teaspoon of Louisiana hot sauce, a cup of chopped celery or a half teaspoon of salt if you like. You can also throw in other vegetables or spices you like with your soup.

2. Cook on "high pressure" setting for 30 minutes. Allow for natural pressure release for 10 minutes and then quick release (QR) the remaining pressure.

3. Remove the ham bone and shred the meat remaining on it back to the soup.

4. Use an immersion blender to roughly puree some of the soup.

5. Serve while hot with some hot sauce on the side.

Recipe Note: *This is a low carb diet, but if you're on a cheat day and are not so strict on low carb you can use pinto beans or dried kidney beans.*

PER SERVING:

Calories: 111 kcal | **Fat:** 1.9g | **Carbs:** 14g | **Protein:** 10g

Chicken Mushroom Soup

This creamy mushroom soup recipe is high in protein and flavor-filled. It is an excellent recipe for your instant pot on the day which you do not have a lot of time for cooking.

TOTAL TIME: 15 MINUTES

SERVINGS: 4

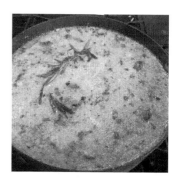

1 lb. skinless and boneless chicken breast in chunks

2 and ½ cups chicken stock

2 cups mushrooms, chopped

3 cloves garlic, minced

1 and ½ cup chopped celery

For Finishing

½ cup full fat coconut milk

1. Make a sauce by blending the garlic with a broth base & coconut milk.

2. Pour the pureed sauce into your instant pots inner liner. Add the chopped celery and chicken breast.

3. Cook the mixture on "high pressure" setting for 5 minutes and then allow for natural pressure release for 10 minutes before you quick release the remaining pressure.

4. Add extra coconut milk (about ½ cup) stir and then serve.

Recipe Notes: *This is an easy creamy chicken soup really. You can throw in just about any of your favorite spices and vegetables.*

PER SERVING:

Calories: 204 kcal | **Fat:** 4g | **Carbs:** 6g | **Protein:** 17g

Low Carb Keto Chicken Noodle Soup

TOTAL TIME: 30 MINUTES

SERVINGS: 2

300 grams Spiral Daikon noodles

2 tsp. Coconut oil

1 b. Chicken thighs (skinned and deboned)

1 cup Celery

1 cup Carrots, diced

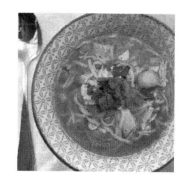

1. In the bowl of your instant pot, add the coconut oil and chicken thighs.

2. Set your instant pot on sauté and timed it for 10 minutes is just enough to have your chicken cooked through.

3. Shred the chicken meat with a fork and add celery and carrots. Remain cooking for another 2 minutes before adding salt to taste.

4. Change the setting to "soup" (timed for 15 minutes). After the timer stops, add daikon noodles and serve.

PER SERVING:

Calories: 371 kcal | **Fat:** 22g | **Carbs:** 6.5g | **Protein:** 36g

Asparagus Soup

TOTAL TIME: 55 MINUTES

SERVINGS: 4

2 lbs. Asparagus, split in half

1 cup Diced ham or 1 ham bone

3 tbsp. Ghee

Salt and seasonings

Onion and minced garlic

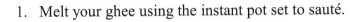

1. Melt your ghee using the instant pot set to sauté.
2. Add onions and garlic and cook for about 5 minutes
3. Add the ham bone or diced ham with salt and seasonings and let it simmer for 2-3 minutes. You may add chicken cube or broth to enhance flavor.
4. Place asparagus and secure your instant pot by sealing and then putting the timer on 45 minutes soup setting.
5. After cooking time completes, allow venting. Take out from the instant pot and blend in a food processor.
6. Serve.

PER SERVING:

Calories: 80 kcal | **Fat:** 2g | **Carbs:** 4g | **Protein:** 6g

Chicken Soup

TOTAL TIME: 10 MINUTES

SERVINGS: 2

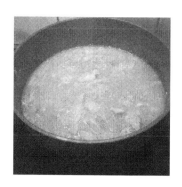

2 Pcs. Chicken breasts, skinned and deboned

2 tbsp. Ghee or butter

1 cup Heavy cream

1/4 cup Onions, diced

1 clove Garlic, minced

1. Combine ingredients except for cream and adjust your instant pot to pressure cooking for 10 minutes. Do a quick vent when the timer is up. Add 3 cups of water or you may use chicken bone-broth instead.
2. Carefully remove the chicken from the pot and place it on a platter to shred chicken meat into pieces using forks. Return it to the pressure cooker and add heavy cream to the soup. Stir to blend ingredients.
3. Serve and enjoy.

PER SERVING:

Calories: 150 kcal | **Fat:** 4g | **Carbs:** 4g | **Protein:** 19g

Quick Onion Soup

TOTAL TIME: 25 MINUTES

SERVINGS: 4

2 tbsp. Avocado oil or coconut oil

8 cups Yellow onions

1 tbsp. Balsamic vinegar

Desired herbs (thyme and bay leaves)

6 cups of pork stock

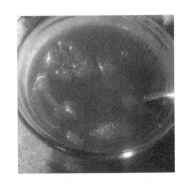

1. Cut onions in half, peel and slice lengthwise.

2. Set instant pot to sauté and then pour oil inside. Add onions and cook, stirring occasionally until they become translucent. This can take about 15 minutes.

3. Add the vinegar and stock, bay leaves, thyme, and salt to taste. Turn off the instant pot and close the lid to secure. For extra caution, check if the float is free, the lid is set on sealing, and the vent isn't blocked.

4. Set the instant pot to high-pressure level and cook the soup for about 10 minutes.

5. Allow pressure to release naturally and never attempt to open the vent as the hot liquid may gush out of it along with the steam.

6. When pressure is totally released, discard the thyme stems and bay leaves and then blend the soup using a blender or if you have an immersion blender, then you can blend it directly into the pot.

7. Serve!

PER SERVING:

Calories: 55 kcal | **Fat:** 1.7g | **Carbs:** 8g | **Protein:** 3.2g

Broccoli Cheddar Soup

TOTAL TIME: 10 MINUTES

SERVINGS: 4

2 heads of fresh broccoli

4 cups Chicken broth

1 cup Heavy Cream

2 cups Cheddar Cheese, shredded

Salt and pepper to taste

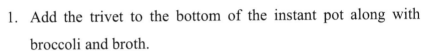

1. Add the trivet to the bottom of the instant pot along with broccoli and broth.
2. Set on manual high pressure for 10 minutes and vent for a quick pressure release. Then remove the trivet and add cream and seasonings.
3. When done, puree in a regular blender and put it back to the instant pot. Add the cheese and heavy cream to melt by stirring.
4. Ladle into bowls and top with desired drips and toppings.

PER SERVING:

Calories: 117 kcal | **Fat:** 8g | **Carbs:** 11g | **Protein:** 3g

Bone Broth

TOTAL TIME: 2 HR 40 MINUTES

SERVINGS: 4

1 lb. bones or bones of one whole organic chicken

2 tbsp. Apple cider vinegar

2 cloves of minced garlic

8 cups water

1 tsp. Sea salt

1. Add all ingredients in an instant pot.
2. Set on soup/brew setting for 2-3 hours. Secure the lid and vent. When done, allow natural pressure release for 10-15 minutes before removing the lid.
3. Strain the liquid and transfer to containers for storing into refrigerators for up to 5 days. For longer storage, store in a freezer instead. Bone soup is healthy and recommended for those with a leaky gut.

PER SERVING:

Calories: 100 kcal | **Fat:** 1g | **Carbs:** 2g | **Protein:** 20g

Instant Pot Dessert Recipes
Creme Brulee

TOTAL TIME: 40 MINUTES

SERVINGS:

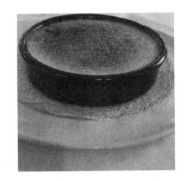

4 cups of heavy cream

1/2 tsp. of sugar

1 tsp. of vanilla extract

1 whole egg

6 egg yolks

1. In a bowl, add the egg, egg yolks, and sugar. Whisk together and whisk until smoothly blended.
2. In a saucepan, heat your heavy cream but don't let boil. Then slowly whisk in the egg mixture into the crème. When thoroughly mixed, remove the pan from the stove and add the vanilla extract. Mix and whisk together.
3. Now, place your trivet inside the instant pot and fill it with 2 cups of water. Prepare your ramekins by spraying the insides with oil. Add in the mixture, about 3/4 full for each ramekin. Then cover the ramekins with foil and arrange them inside the instant pot on top of the trivet. Cook in batches (about 4 ramekins for each batch).
4. Once in place, secure the vent, close the lid cover and set it to manual mode. Set the timer for 11 minutes. Once the timer goes off, do a quick pressure release and when you are able

to open the instant pot, gently place the ramekins on a cookie sheet and allow to cook for 30 minutes.

5. Place them in the fridge for about two hours to chill. Just leave the foil on especially when you cool them overnight. Once ready to serve, sprinkle some sugar on top of each ramekin and give each a shake. Then caramelize the top using a torch or you may use your oven and set it to broil mode, but make sure they don't get burned.

PER SERVING:

Calories: 210 kcal | **Fat:** 10g | **Carbs:** 18g | **Protein:** 13g

Spiced Cider

TOTAL TIME: 25 MINUTES

SERVINGS: 4

5-6 Organic apples, unpeeled

2 Cinnamon sticks

1 pc. Organic ginger, peeled

2 cloves garlic

1 tbsp. Maple syrup

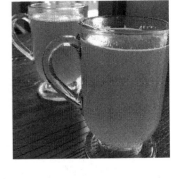

1. Clean and core the apple but do not peel. Place them in a blender with water up to the level of the 4 cups marking.
2. Puree the apples until well-blended and then let the mixture pass through a strainer before pouring it into the instant pot.
3. Using a spoon, release as much water out of the apple pulp as you much as you can, so you have to repeat the process several times.
4. Place the stainless pot inside filled with water up to 6 cups (refer to the mark on the inside portion of the pot.
5. Add cinnamon sticks, cloves, and ginger along with the maple syrup.
6. Secure the valve by sealing and set the pot on manual (high) mode for 13 minutes.
7. Once it beeps, allow the pressure to release in a natural manner for 10 minutes before carefully opening the lid cover.
8. Stir lightly and then ladle into mugs for serving.

PER SERVING:

Calories: 80 kcal | **Fat:** 0g | **Carbs:** 20g | **Protein:** 0g

Ricotta Lemon Cheesecake

TOTAL TIME: 30 MINUTES

SERVINGS: 1

1/3 cup Ricotta cheese

1/2 tsp. Lemon extract from a lemon, lemon juice, and zest

2 eggs

2 tbsp. Sour cream

1 tbsp. Stevia (sweetener)

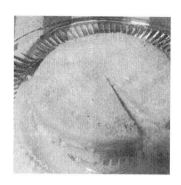

1. Combine ingredients except for eggs in a standing mixer bowl and mix until you arrive at a smooth mixture consistency without lumps.
2. Taste to make sure that the sweetness is according to your taste.
3. Crack 2 eggs while reducing the speed of the mixer and gently bend until the egg is thoroughly mixed with the rest of the ingredients. However, make sure that you don't overbeat at this stage as it will result in a cracker crust.
4. Pour the mixture into a 6-inch greased spring-form pan and cover it with foil and silicone lid.
5. In your instant pot, place the trivet and add two cups of water. Place the foil-covered pan on top of the trivet.
6. Cook on high pressure for 30 minutes, allowing pressure to release naturally.

7. Mix sour cream with Stevia and spread over the warm cake.

8. Refrigerate the cheesecake for 6-8 hours before serving.

PER SERVING:

Calories: 300 kcal | **Fat:** 21g | **Carbs:** 25g | **Protein:** 17g

Coconut Yogurt

TOTAL TIME: 8 HR

SERVINGS: 4

3 14-oz. cans of refrigerated, coconut milk

2 tbsp. Gelatine

1 tbsp. Honey or maple syrup

4 Probiotics capsules

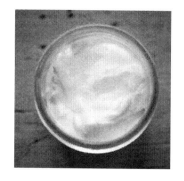

1. Remove the solid cream on top of the coconut milk and transfer it to the instant bow.

2. Secure the lid by sealing the vent then press the yogurt button. Next, adjust to BOIL.

3. When the process is completed, the pot will prompt you by beeping. Remove the bowl from the pot and leave to cool.

4. Use a thermometer to see if the mixture had reached 100 degrees Fahrenheit or 38 degrees Centigrade. This is to ensure that the culture is active.

5. Open the probiotics capsule and slowly whisk its content into the coconut cream.

6. Put the bowl back into the instant pot and close the lid. Press YOGURT and then press the plus sign (+) to set the time for about 8 hours.

7. In a blender, add the yogurt and slowly mix in the gelatin while blending. This is to thicken the consistency of the

yogurt. Then add additionally desired flavoring such as vanilla, honey, etc.)

8. Store in the fridge for a few hours to set and cool.

PER SERVING:

Calories: 140 kcal | **Fat:** 6g | **Carbs:** 22g | **Protein:** 1g

Low Carb Peanut Butter Chocolate Cheesecake

TOTAL TIME: 20 MINUTES

SERVINGS: 2

16 Oz. Cream cheese

2 tbsp. Powdered peanut butter

2 pcs. Eggs, large

1 tbsp. Cocoa

1/2 cup Sugar substitute

1. Ensure that all ingredients are at room temperature.
2. Add eggs and cream cheese to a blender and blend until smooth.
3. Add the rest of the ingredients and thoroughly blend.
4. Put the well-blended mixture into a 4 or 8-ounce mason jars and put a foil or lid cover.
5. Add a cup of water to the instant pot and also, put inside it the trivet.
6. Arrange the jars inside the instant pot on top of the trivet and cook in batches.
7. Set on high pressure for 15-18 minute and allow it to naturally release pressure.
8. Chill for a few hours or overnight.
9. Topped with whipped heavy cream and with peanut butter or you may add a few chopped peanuts to add texture.

PER SERVING:

Calories: 410 kcal | **Fat:** 24g | **Carbs:** 12.5g | **Protein:** 10g

Baked Apples

TOTAL TIME: 4 MINUTES

SERVINGS: 4

4 pcs of medium-size apples

2 tsp. Cinnamon

2 tsp. Honey

1/2 cup Water

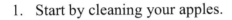

1. Start by cleaning your apples.
2. Cut apples into slices and remove all seeds.
3. Combine all the ingredients including apples, cinnamon, honey, and water in the instant pot and toss.
4. Secure the lid of the instant pot by setting the vent to seal and turn to manual mode setting for 2 minutes.
5. When the timer goes off, open the valve for quick release of pressure. Allow all pressure to be released compete. Once the pressure is completely released, toss the apples once again and serve.

PER SERVING:

Calories: 268 kcal | **Fat:** 4g | **Carbs:** 60g | **Protein:** 0.3g

BONUS:
5 Day Ultimate Ketogenic Meal Plan for Rapid Fat Loss

First of all, I would like to thank you from the bottom of my heart for trusting and giving me an opportunity to hold your hand and go the extra mile with you. I hope to be part of every journey you take, guiding you along the path towards your goals. Once again, thank you for your support and if you find this book somehow interesting, which I really hope you do :P. Please do sacrifice a minute of your precious time and take a look at my previous published eBooks which hit the top lists of both Amazon's #1 & #2 Best Selling eBooks with Images! Right now, I'm going to share with you a 5 Day Ketogenic Meal Plan for Breakfast, Lunch & Dinner. For full version, please check out: https://www.amazon.com/dp/B01MR01ELG

Without further ado, let's get started!

FIRST WEEK	BREAKFAST	LUNCH	DINNER
Monday	Cheesy Jalapeno Egg Muffins	Stir-Fried Shrimps with Asparagus and Snap Pea	Chicken Gumbo
Tuesday	Coconut Flour Waffles	Honey-Soy Sesame Chicken	Oven-Baked Spinach and Quinoa
Wednesday	Low-Carb Breakfast Patties	Mongolian Beef	Tomato-Mushroom Chicken Casserole
Thursday	Cheesy Spinach and Mushroom Quiche	Chicken and Broccoli Stir-Fry	Black Bean and Chickpea Soup with Chorizo
Friday	Sausage and Spinach Mini Cups	Salmon Fillets with Curry Sauce and Cucumbers	Lemon-Peppered Prawns

Breakfast Recipes

Cheesy Jalapeno Egg Muffins

Preparation time: 10 minutes
Cooking time: 25 to 30 minutes
Serves: 4

Ingredients:
- 8 strips of bacon
- 8 free-range eggs
- ½ cup of grated sharp Cheddar cheese
- ¼ cup of softened cream cheese
- 4 green jalapeno peppers, thinly sliced
- ¼ teaspoon of garlic powder
- ¼ teaspoon of onion powder
- Sea salt and black pepper, as needed to taste
- Coconut or olive oil, for greasing

Directions:
1. Preheat oven to 375°F. Lightly grease a muffin tray with oil and set aside.
2. In a pan over medium-high heat, add the bacon and cook until lightly crisp but still pliable. Remove the bacon from the pan, transfer into a plate with paper towels and reserve the bacon fat.
3. Combine the eggs, cream cheese, jalapeno peppers, onion powder, garlic powder and bacon grease in a mixing bowl and mix until the ingredients are well incorporated. Season it with salt and black pepper and mix to combine, set aside.
4. Place 1 to 1 ½ strips of bacon on the sides of the muffin tins and pour in the egg mixture. Fill each tin about ¾ full only. Top with shredded cheddar cheese and sliced jalapenos.

Cook it in the oven for about 20 to 25 minute, or until the cheese has melted and lightly browned.
5. Remove from the oven, transfer into a wire rack and let it rest for about 5 minutes before serving. Remove egg muffins from tray, transfer into a serving platter and serve immediately.

Nutrition Facts (per serving):

Kcal 201.8	Protein 17.5 g	Fat 16 g
Carbs 3.34 g	Fiber 1.3 g	Sugar 0.5 g

Coconut Flour Waffles

Preparation time: 10 minutes
Cooking time: 5 to 10 minutes
Serves: 4

Ingredients:

- 6 medium free range whole eggs
- ¼ cup of grass-fed butter or coconut oil
- 1 teaspoon of raw cane sugar
- ½ teaspoon of fine sea salt
- ½ teaspoon of baking powder
- ½ cup sifted coconut flour
- Oil, for greasing

Directions:

1. Whisk together the ghee and eggs in a mixing bowl until well combined.
2. In a separate large bowl, add the flour, stevia, salt and baking powder and then mix it thoroughly until well incorporated. Pour in the egg mixture and mix it well until smooth and the ingredients are evenly distributed. Let it rest for about 10 minutes to let the mixture rise.
3. Preheat a waffle maker and lightly grease with oil. Once the waffle maker plate is hot, add the mixture and cook according to the appliance directions.
4. Remove the waffles, divide into 4 equal portions and serve warm.

Nutrition Facts (per serving):

Kcal 366	Protein 17.5 g	Fat 25.8g
Carbs 4.25 g	Fiber 2.75 g	Sugar 1 g

Low-Carb Breakfast Patties

Preparation time: 5 minutes
Cooking time: 10 minutes
Serves: 4 to 6

Ingredients:
- 1 cup of almond or coconut flour
- 2 large free-range eggs
- ½ cup of heavy cream
- ½ cup melted grass-fed unsalted butter
- 1 teaspoon of vanilla extract or syrup
- ½ teaspoon of baking soda
- 8 slices of turkey bacon
- ¼ cup of water

Directions:
1. In a pan over medium-high heat, add the bacon and cook until crisp. Remove from the pan reserving the bacon fat, transfer into plate with paper towels and chop the bacon into small pieces.
2. In a mixing bowl, whisk together the egg, cream, melted butter, vanilla syrup and water until well incorporated. Set aside.
3. In a separate mixing bowl, combine together the flour and baking soda until well combined. Pour in the egg mixture and mix until smooth and the ingredients are evenly distributed.
4. In the same pan with bacon fat, apply medium-high heat and pour in about 1/8 of the batter mixture. Swirl the pan to fully coat the bottom with the batter and sprinkle with chopped bacon on top. Cook the pancake for about 3 to 4 minutes on each side, or until the bottom is lightly browned. Flip it over to cook the other side for another 3 to 4 minutes. Repeat the procedure with the remaining batter mixture.
5. Transfer into a serving platter and serve immediately.

Nutrition Facts (per serving):

Kcal 259.5	Protein 7.5 g	Fat 3.5 g
Carbs 3.25 g	Fiber 1.5 g	Sugar 0.75 g

Cheesy Spinach and Mushroom Quiche

Preparation time: 15 minutes
Cooking time: 45 minutes
Serves: 4 to 6

Ingredients:

- ½ pound of fresh mushrooms, sliced
- ½ teaspoon minced garlic
- 1 cup of chopped spinach
- 4 large free range whole eggs
- 1 cup of whole milk
- ¼ cup of crumbled Feta cheese
- ¼ cup of grated Parmesan cheese
- ½ cup shredded Mozzarella cheese
- Salt and ground black pepper, to taste

Directions:

1. Preheat an oven to 350°F and lightly grease a pie dish and set aside.
2. In a skillet over medium-high heat, lightly coat the bottom with oil and sauté the mushrooms until soft. Stir in the garlic and season to taste with salt and pepper. Sauté for about 5 to 6 minutes while stirring occasionally.
3. While sautéing the mushrooms, add the milk, eggs, grated Parmesan in separate mixing bowl and whisk until well combined. Season with salt and pepper and briefly mix to combine. Set aside.
4. Place the spinach evenly on the bottom of the prepared pie dish and place the sautéed mushrooms on top. Add the crumbled feta cheese evenly on top of the mushrooms and pour in the egg mixture. Add the shredded Mozzarella cheese evenly over the egg mixture, place it on a baking sheet and bake it in the oven for about 40 to 45 minutes or until the center is set and cooked through.

5. Remove from the oven, transfer on a wire rack and let it rest for about 5 minutes before serving. Slice into 6 equal portions and serve immediately.
6. Spray a pie dish with non-stick spray. Squeeze the rest of the water out of the spinach and spread it out on the bottom of the pie dish. Next, add the cooked mushrooms and crumbled feta.

Nutrition Facts (per serving):

Kcal 172.5	Protein 20 g	Fat 10.5 g
Carbs 5.8 g	Fiber 1 g	Sugar 3.2 g

Sausage and Spinach Mini Cups

Preparation time: 15 minutes
Cooking time: 30 minutes
Serves: 4

Ingredients:
- 1 cup of chopped spinach, blanched ahead
- 4 links of smoked pork sausage, cooked ahead, casing removed and chopped
- 1 large sweet green pepper, deseeded and minced
- 1 medium yellow onion, minced
- ½ cup of shredded sharp Cheddar cheese
- 5 large free range whole eggs
- ¼ cup heavy whipping cream, whipped
- ½ teaspoon of garlic powder
- ½ teaspoon of onion powder
- ½ teaspoon of ground black pepper
- ½ teaspoon of real sea salt
- 1 cup of cherry tomatoes
- Oil, for greasing

Directions:
1. Preheat oven to 350°F and lightly grease a muffin tray with oil and set aside.
2. Lightly coat a skillet with oil and apply with medium-high heat. Add the minced pepper and onions, and then sauté for about 3 minutes or until the vegetables are soft and tender. Stir in the cooked sausage and spinach and cook for about 2 minutes or until warmed through. Remove pan from heat and let it rest to cool.
3. In a large mixing bowl, whisk together the eggs, cream, garlic powder, onion powder, black pepper and salt until well combined. Mix in the Cheddar cheese and sautéed

4. spinach-sausage mixture into the bowl and mix it thoroughly until well incorporated.
5. Add the mixture evenly on each muffin cup and top with one cherry tomato. Bake it in the oven for about 20 to 30 minutes or until the center is set and cooked through. Remove from the oven, transfer into a wire rack and let it rest for about 5 minutes before serving.
6. Remove the muffins from the tray, transfer into a serving platter and serve immediately.

Nutrition Facts (per serving):

Kcal 213.9	Protein 15.9 g	Fat 17.5 g
Carbs 3.4 g	Fiber .8 g	Sugar .2 g

Lunch Recipes

Stir-Fried Shrimps with Asparagus and Snap Pea

Preparation time: 5 minutes
Cooking time: 15 minutes
Serves: 4

Ingredients:
- ½ pound fresh asparagus spears, trimmed and cut into bias
- 1 pound of fresh shrimp, peeled and deveined
- 2 tablespoons of coconut or olive oil
- 1 teaspoon minced fresh ginger root
- 2 teaspoons minced garlic
- 1 red sweet peppers, sliced into strips
- 1 medium onion, sliced into thin strips
- ½ pound fresh yellow snap peas
- 1 teaspoon sesame seeds
- 2 tablespoons light soy sauce (or namu shoyu)
- 2 tablespoons finely chopped coriander
- 2 tablespoons toasted sesame oil

Directions:
1. In a wok over medium-high heat, add the oil and heat until it starts to smoke. Add the garlic and ginger, cook for 20 seconds while stirring constantly. Add the shrimp and cook it until the color turns opaque. Stir in the asparagus, bell pepper, snap peas and onion in the wok and cook for 4 minutes, or until the vegetables are soft while stirring occasionally.
2. Stir in the soy sauce, sesame oil and coriander and gently toss to coat. Remove wok from heat.
3. Transfer into individual serving plates and serve warm with extra lemon wedges, if preferred.

Nutrition Facts (per serving)

Kcal 306	Protein 27.5 g	Fat 13.5 g
Carbs 10.75 g	Fiber 5.75 g	Sugar 4.75 g

Honey-Soy Sesame Chicken

Preparation time: 5 minutes
Cooking time: 20 to 25 minutes
Serves: 4

Ingredients:

- 2 free-range chicken breast (skinless and boneless), cut into 1-inch strips
- ¼ cup of raw honey
- ¼ cup of light soy sauce
- ½ cup of chicken stock or water
- 2 tablespoons of arrowroot starch
- 2 tablespoon coconut or olive oil
- 1 teaspoon of grated fresh ginger root
- ½ crushed red pepper flakes (optional)
- 1 teaspoon sesame seeds, toasted

Directions:

1. In a skillet over medium-high heat, add the oil and heat until it starts to smoke. Add the chicken and cook for 6 minutes, or until lightly brown.
2. In a mixing bowl, combine the soy sauce, honey, water, arrowroot starch, ginger and pepper flakes. Whisk thoroughly until dissolved completely.
3. Add the sauce mixture in the skillet and cook for about 5 to 6 minutes while stirring occasionally. Sprinkle in the sesame seeds and add more water if the sauce is too thick.
4. Cover with lid and cook for another 10 minutes with medium-low heat. Transfer into serving dishes and serve warm.

Nutrition Facts (per serving)

Kcal 264	Protein 30.5 g	Fat 12.5 g
Carbs 9.5 g	Fiber .5 g	Sugar 9 g

Mongolian Beef

Preparation time: 10 minutes
Cooking time: 20 minutes
Serves: 4

Ingredients:

- 2 tablespoons of coconut oil
- 2 teaspoons minced fresh ginger root
- 1 teaspoon minced garlic
- ¼ cup light soy sauce or namu shoyu
- ¼ cup of beef stock or water
- ¼ cup of raw cane sugar
- 1 tablespoon olive oil, or as needed for frying
- 1 pound of grass-fed beef flank steaks, trimmed and sliced into thin strips
- ¼ cup coconut flour or arrowroot flour
- ¼ tablespoon red pepper flakes (optional)
- 2 medium stems of green onions, cut on the bias

Directions:

1. Coat all sides of the beef evenly with flour, place on a plate and set aside.
2. In a saucepan over medium-high heat, add in the olive oil. When the oil is hot, sauté the garlic and ginger for 30 seconds while stirring constantly. Stir in the soy sauce and sugar, bring to a boil and cook until the sauce has thickened. Remove pan from heat and set aside.
3. In a separate pan over medium-high heat, add 1 tablespoon of oil and fry half of the beef for 3 minutes or until browned. Remove from pan with a slotted spoon and cook the remaining beef for another 3 minutes. Stir the meat constantly to cook it evenly on all sides. Remove from pan, discard the oil and return the beef into the pan.

4. Pour in the sauce, cook for about 3 to 4 minutes while stirring regularly. Add the red pepper flakes and bring to a boil. Remove pan from heat.
5. Transfer the beef into individual serving plates, pour with sauce and top with green onions. Serve immediately.

Nutrition Facts (per serving)

Kcal 333.4	Protein 26 g	Fat 15.5 g
Carbs 9 g	Fiber 1.5 g	Sugar 8 g

Chicken and Broccoli Stir-Fry

Preparation time: 5 minutes
Cooking time: 20 minutes
Serves: 4

Ingredients:
- ½ cup of water or chicken stock
- 3 to 4 tablespoons of light soy sauce or namu shoyu
- 1 pound of detached broccoli florets
- 2 teaspoons arrowroot starch
- 2 tablespoons of hoisin sauce
- 1 teaspoon minced fresh ginger root
- ½ tablespoon sesame oil
- 1 large yellow bell pepper, sliced into thin strips
- 2 tablespoons olive or coconut oil
- 4 free-range chicken breast fillets, cut into cubes

Directions:
1. Whisk together the water, soy sauce, corn starch, ginger, hoisin sauce and sesame oil in a bowl until well combined. Set aside.
2. In a wok, add half of the oil and apply medium-high heat. Cook the broccoli florets and bell peppers for 3 to 4 minutes, or until the vegetables are soft and season with salt and pepper. Remove vegetables from wok, transfer on a plate and set aside.
3. On the same wok, add the remaining oil and apply medium-high heat. Add the chicken and cook until brown, for about 3 minutes. Add in the sauce mixture and gently toss to coat the chicken evenly. Return the broccoli and bell peppers, cook for 2 minutes while stirring regularly. Remove skillet from heat.

4. Portion the chicken and broccoli on individual serving plates, pour over the sauce and serve warm with toasted sesame on top.

Nutrition Facts (per serving)

Kcal 378	Protein 25.5 g	Fat 14.8 g
Carbs 6.25 g	Fiber 5.25 g	Sugar 4.5 g

Salmon Fillets with Curry Sauce and Cucumbers

Preparation time: 15 minutes
Cooking time: 10 minutes
Serves: 4

Ingredients:

- 1 cucumbers, preferably seedless, sliced
- 4 (4 oz.) skinless wild-caught salmon fillets
- ¼ cup of red curry paste
- 2 tablespoons of coconut or olive oil
- 1 large organic lemon, juiced
- 1 medium spring onion, chopped
- 2 teaspoons minced garlic
- 1-inch piece of fresh ginger root, minced
- 1 red hot chilli pepper, finely chopped
- Salt and black pepper, to taste
- Small bunch cilantro, roughly chopped

Directions:

1. Apply with medium-high heat on a pan and the oil when it is hot. When the oil is hot, add the onions, garlic, chili and ginger and then sauté for 2 minutes or until fragrant. Stir in the curry paste and half of the chopped cilantro and sauté for about 2 minutes while stirring occasionally.
2. Season the salmon with salt and pepper on both sides and place it in the pan. Add the lemon juice and chilli pepper and baste the fillets with sauce to cover. Cover with lid and cook for about 8 to 10 minutes.
3. Place the cucumbers on a serving bowl, carefully remove the fillets from the pan and transfer it on top of the cucumbers. Pour the sauce over the salmon and cucumbers, and then serve immediately with chopped spring onions and the remaining cilantro on top.

Nutrition Facts (per serving):

Kcal 195.5	Protein 24.5 g	Fat 8.25 g
Carbs 7.25 g	Fiber .75 g	Sugar 3.25 g

Dinner Recipes

Chicken Gumbo

Preparation time: 5 minutes
Cooking time: 25 minutes
Serves: 4 to 6

Ingredients:
- 2 tablespoons olive oil
- ¼ cup almond or coconut flour
- 2 diced bell peppers
- 1 red onion, diced
- 2 teaspoons minced garlic
- 1 ½ teaspoons dried oregano
- Salt and ground black pepper, to taste
- ½ pound of fresh okra, base-trimmed
- 2 medium links of smoked sausage, halved and finely chopped
- 1 ½ pounds of precooked chicken meat, shredded

Directions:
1. In a large pot over medium-high heat, add in the oil. Stir in the flour, and then cook until lightly golden while stirring constantly. Stir in the bell peppers, garlic, onions and oregano in the pot. Cook it for about 5 to 7 minutes, or until the vegetables are soft and aromatic.
2. Pour in 750 ml of water and add the sausage and okra. Cover lid and bring the liquid mixture to a boil. Add the chicken and season to taste with pepper and salt. Cook for 2 minutes while stirring regularly, or until warmed through. Remove pot from heat.
3. Portion chicken gumbo on individual serving bowls. Serve immediately.

Nutrition Facts (per serving)

Kcal 301	Protein 22.75 g	Fat 17.5 g
Carbs 12.1 g	Fiber 2 g	Sugar 2.7 g

Oven-Baked Spinach and Quinoa

Preparation time: 5 minutes
Cooking time: 25 minutes
Serves: 4

Ingredients:
- 1 cup of rinsed and drained quinoa
- 1 cup of chicken stock
- 2 tablespoons of olive or coconut oil
- 2 cups packed fresh baby spinach
- 1 cup of unsweetened almond or coconut milk
- 1 to 2 free-range eggs
- ¼ teaspoon of real sea salt
- ¼ teaspoon ground pepper
- ½ cup of grated Mozzarella or Cheddar cheese

Directions:
1. Preheat oven to 350°F.
2. Bring the chicken broth to a boil in a large saucepan. Add the quinoa and simmer, covered, for 15 to 20 minutes, until quinoa is tender and liquid is absorbed.
3. Meanwhile, in a large skillet, heat the oil over medium heat. Add the spinach and sauté just for about 1 to 2 minutes, or until slightly wilted.
4. Stir the sautéed spinach into the cooked quinoa. Whisk together the milk, egg, salt and pepper in a small bowl. Add milk mixture and half the cheese to the quinoa mixture and stir well.
5. Transfer to a lightly greased casserole dish and bake, uncovered, for 30 minutes. Sprinkle with the remaining 125 g cheese and bake until melted, about 5 more minutes. Serve.

Nutrition Facts (per serving)

Kcal 328.75	Protein 24.25g	Fat 15.25 g
Carbs 14.75 g	Fiber 3.25 g	Sugar 4.5 g

Tomato-Mushroom Chicken Casserole

Preparation time: 5 minutes
Cooking time: 25 minutes
Serves: 4

Ingredients:
- 1 cup of chicken broth
- ½ cup grated sharp Cheddar cheese
- ½ cup softened cream cheese
- 1 cup cream of mushroom soup
- 1 cup of canned stewed tomatoes
- ½ teaspoon crushed red pepper flakes
- 1 pound precooked chicken meat, cubed
- 4 medium rounds of corn tortillas
- 2 tablespoons coconut or olive oil
- Black pepper, to taste

Directions:
1. Preheat an oven to a temperature of 350°F. Lightly grease a casserole with oil and set aside.
2. In a pan over medium-high heat, add 1 tablespoon of oil and reheat the chicken for about 1 to 2 minutes. Remove from heat and transfer to a bowl. Set aside.
3. In a large mixing bowl, combine the cream of chicken, cream of mushroom, and the stewed tomatoes with its juice. Stir in the cream cheese and red pepper flakes, add the chicken and season with black pepper. Gently stir to combine and set aside.
4. Place the corn tortillas on the prepared casserole and make sure to fully cover the bottom, pour in the chicken mixture and spread evenly on the casserole using a spatula. Top with grated cheddar cheese and bake it in the oven for about 20 to 25 minutes, or until the chicken is thoroughly cooked and the cheese has melted.

5. Remove the casserole from the oven, transfer on a wire rack and let it rest for 5 minutes before serving.

Nutrition Facts (per serving)

Kcal 328	Protein 36 g	Fat 15.75 g
Carbs 11 g	Fiber 2.75 g	Sugar 3 g

Black Bean and Chickpea Soup with Chorizo

Preparation time: 5 minutes
Cooking time: 20 to 25 minutes
Serves: 4

Ingredients:

- 2 tablespoon of coconut or olive oil, divided
- ¾ cup of canned black beans, drained and mashed
- ½ cup canned chickpeas, drained
- 1 large red onion, diced
- 1 medium red bell pepper, diced
- 1 medium green bell pepper, diced
- 1 teaspoon minced fresh oregano
- 1 teaspoon minced garlic
- 1 large pinch of cumin powder
- ½ teaspoon chili powder
- ¼ teaspoon salt
- 3 to 4 cups of chicken stock
- 4 medium links of smoked pork chorizo, casings-removed and chopped
- ¼ cup of sour cream, for serving (optional)
- Chopped fresh cilantro, for serving

Directions:

1. In a large saucepan over medium heat, add in half of the olive oil. Once the oil is hot, add the chorizo and cook for 3 to 4 minutes or until lightly brown. Remove chorizo from pan with a slotted spoon, transfer on a plate and set aside.
2. In the same pan, add the remaining oil and sauté the onions and bell pepper for 3 minutes, or until the vegetables are soft. Stir in the garlic, chili powder, salt, beans, and chickpea and then pour in the stock. Cover lid and bring to a boil. Reduce to low heat, stir in the chorizo and simmer for 5 minutes.

3. Remove from heat and portion soup into individual serving bowls. Serve warm with sour cream and chopped cilantro on top.

Nutrition Facts (per serving)

Kcal 434	Protein 22.75 g	Fat 18.5 g
Carbs 8.5 g	Fiber 11.5 g	Sugar 5.25 g

Lemon-Peppered Prawns

Preparation time: 5 minutes
Cooking time: 10 minutes
Serves: 4

Ingredients:
- 1 ½ pounds of fresh prawns, peeled and deveined
- 2 to 3 tablespoons of coconut oil
- 2 medium stems of spring onion, thinly sliced

For the Marinade:
- 1 teaspoon of minced garlic
- 2 medium lemons, juiced and zested
- 1 teaspoon of freshly cracked black peppercorns
- Real sea salt, as needed to taste

Directions:
1. Add all marinade ingredients in a large bowl and mix until well combined. Add the prawns and gently toss to evenly coat with the marinade mixture. Cover the bowl with plastic wrap and marinate for at least 2 hours.
2. In a non-stick skillet or pan, apply high heat and add the oil. Once the oil is hot, add the prawns and cook for about 5 to 6 minutes while stirring regularly. Cook until the color turns opaque and remove the skillet from heat.
3. Add the spring onions and gently toss to combine. Transfer into a serving platter and serve immediately with extra lemon wedges, if desired.

Nutrition Facts (per serving)

Kcal 133.25	Protein 23.5 g	Fat 12 g
Carbs 3.75 g	Fiber .75 g	Sugar .55 g

Conclusion

When the government, NGOs, and private sectors are working hard to spread health awareness among the people in order to counter the alarming increase of deadly diseases, diets and physical fitness became a trend. Most of these diets and physical training are geared towards weight loss in the hope of fighting against obesity which has become a common health risk for these deadly diseases.

When most diets aim to reduce calorie consumption and get away from fat, Ketogenic diet seems to work contrary to these conventional food diets. It focuses on increasing fat consumption while reducing calorie.

Preparing and cooking a ketogenic meal is great and healthy, but when you are on a tight budget or don't have enough time to prepare a complicated meal, then that's where you can benefit from the technology of a multi-cooking gadget needed in every home.

When this useful kitchen gadget can help you manage your time in the kitchen with absolutely no hassles to panic over meal timings, then cooking can be both fun and exciting especially for mothers who seem to be always in a constant rush when it comes to mealtimes.

With the Instant Pot, there's no need to trouble yourself with cleaning too many pots and pans since it's a multi-cooker in one. You can cook rice, sauté, pressure cook, slow cook, and steam in just one pot! Just press the buttons according to what you want your Instant Pot to do for you and whoa! It's done quicker than the conventional way of cooking.

Combining the benefits of ketogenic diet and an instant pot is indeed a kitchen revolution!

-- GEN GALE

Check out Other Best Selling eBooks

Quick & Easy Metabolism Miracle Diet:
Shed Stubborn Fats With 5 Ingredients Or Less

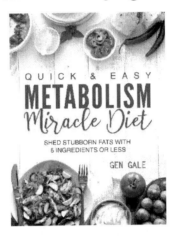

Amazon's #1 Best Seller:
https://www.amazon.com/dp/B074CDRFLS

The Ultimate Ketogenic Lifestyle:
14 Day Fat Burning, Delicious Low Carb Recipes for Breakfast, Lunch & Dinner

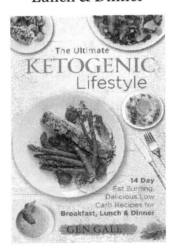

Amazon's #2 Best Seller:
https://www.amazon.com/dp/B01MR01ELG

What Makes Us Fat:
Change Your Lifestyle In 7 Days

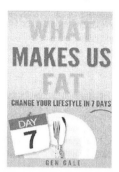

https://www.amazon.com/dp/B01N3UWOYX

Made in the USA
Lexington, KY
28 March 2018